Dear Friend

Thirty days to healing

Ronald E. Kearns

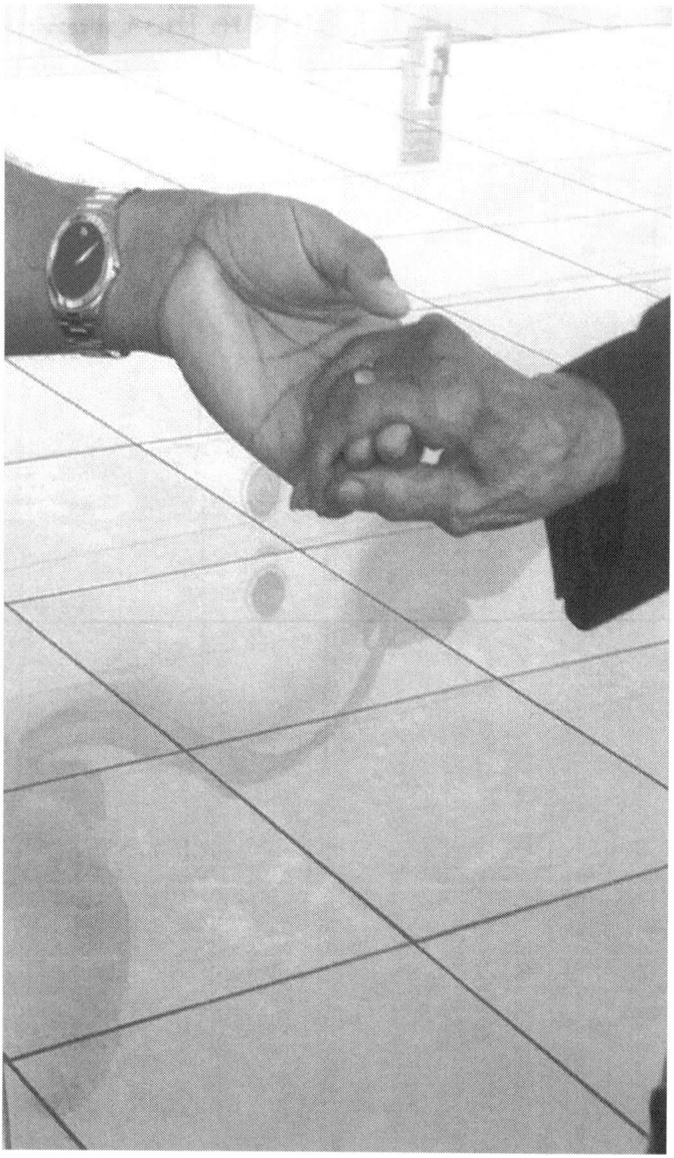

Dedicated to the memory of Lillie B. Kearns

Purpose

The purpose of this book is to help readers through the grieving process. Years ago when my father died the pastor gave each member of my immediate family a copy of the book Good Grief by Granger Westberg, Fortress Press. That book was very helpful for me to identify the stages of grief.

When my wife died in 2019, I re-read the book to help me through the grieving process once again. After reading it I kept a journal to express what I was feeling and how I was dealing with it. While reading through my journal I discovered that others going through the grieving process could benefit from what I went through. Along with Good Grief and other books on grief I think that this book from someone grieving can help.

I suggest that anyone grieving seeks counseling if only for a brief time. It's important to openly discuss your feelings with someone who can help you process them. It's very important that you know that you are not alone in your feelings nor are you the first person to experience those feelings. It's normal to grieve whether you do it openly or behind closed doors. You must learn how to acknowledge your pain.

Everything discussed in the book may not apply to you but there are things we all experience. The main thing we all experience is change. Things won't be the same based on the absence of the source of our grief. Whether we're grieving a person or a pet the sense of loss is .the same. I would recommend reading only one letter a day to give yourself a chance to process what you have read. Psalm 30:5 ...weeping may stay for the night, but Joy comes in the morning. I strongly suggest that you read one letter a day and take time to process and digest what you have read.

Dear Friend,

The first emotion or feeling you go through is probably shock. How did this happen? Why did this happen? Why did this happen to us? Shock is a normal reaction even if our loved one has battled a disease for a long time. We are never prepared for loss. Probably the most difficult part of loss is that we encounter a sudden change in life as we know it. Adjusting to change is difficult even in the best of circumstances but change brought on by death can seem insurmountable.

What can I do? How can I go on? Those two questions are questions we each ask in some form. During the preparations for the funeral or memorial service you will keep busy at first and having friends or loved ones around can shield us for a while. But in our quiet alone moments those two questions loom heavy on our spirits. Some people hide from the questions and retreat inward closing themselves off from reality and others. Some people thrust themselves into various activities. Neither of those is healthy if you're evading the issue at hand.

As difficult as it may be, you have to address your future without your loved one. There will be overwhelming sadness at first. It would be abnormal if you didn't feel the loss. I discovered I had to consciously decide to go on with life because that was what my wife would've wanted. For forty-nine years my life was centered around "us." Suddenly, I was plunged into a situation where my future was built around "me."

I had to learn how to navigate life as a widower, a title I had never imagined. Shock was a reaction to the loss but I could not allow it to shape my life. I had to accept the fact that my wife's life had ended but mine had to go on. Bills still had to be paid, meals had to be prepared and I still had to go about every day activities. As much as I may have wanted to curl up and let life go on without me that was not healthy and I needed to move on. You must want to change even though it will be difficult.

Love,

Ron

Dear Friend,

You may have awakened this morning overwhelmed by a sense of loss. You may ask why did you have to suffer this loss. It may have been difficult for you to just pull yourself out of bed. You're experiencing an early stage of grief. What I want you to know is that this is natural. Grieving is to be expected when you suffer loss.

The problem a lot of people have is trying to suppress grieving and hold back the emotions. I never allowed myself to hold in my emotions. For me, releasing helped me have enough strength to deal with my grief. The analogy I use is a teapot with a steam whistle. As the steam in the tiny teapot accumulates the more the pressure builds and it becomes more likely the teapot is going to implode or explode. The steam whistle allows the steam to release without damage to the teapot. The same is true about the human body. If we try to hold in grief the pressure builds. Implosion means a heart attack, a stroke or any number of health problems. Explosion means verbally or physically attacking people. The pressure will be released whether little by little or one great burst. Crying is not something to be ashamed of. It's how your body releases the pressure that's built up. Don't fight it. Find a private place where you can release. For me it's my bedroom or bathroom. I may cry softly or loudly however my grief manifests itself. Once again, I learned early on not to attempt to hold it in. Love,

Ron

Dear Friend,

It's natural when we experience loss to question "why me." The reason we grieve is because we take loss personally. This is a part of the grieving process but you can't allow yourself to get lost in this stage of grieving. Was the person we loss in pain? Were they suffering greatly? Are we being selfish because what we're going through is more important than their being out of pain and suffering? Did they die suddenly without warning? Is it more about us than it is about them?

These are questions we must ask ourselves in order to get beyond this stage. Did we enjoy watching them suffer? Of course we didn't. We would've preferred that they be healed or helped immediately. Since that didn't happen we have to deal with the outcome. When I was younger I didn't understand why adults cried when they loss a parent.

After all, they were old, why were you surprised they died? My father, a pastor, explained to me that no matter how long you had your parents you wanted them longer. Age has nothing to do with how we grieve. Gender has nothing to do with how we grieve. As a boy society taught me that men don't cry. I saw my father, one of the strongest men I've ever known, cry when his mother died. I learned at that moment that real men cry.

You can't buy into the lie that crying is a weakness. Releasing by crying has given me strength. I have felt stronger and more able to face adversity after crying. I find a quiet place for reflection and meditation to release. Interestingly enough, I have more energy after crying. I'm not suggesting that crying is the only way to release. As a musician I play my grief out. My instrument becomes my voice. For you it may be swimming or playing sports. It may be drawing or painting. It may be long runs or long

13

walks. My point is, allow yourself to find a way to regroup and find your new normal. Don't allow others to dictate how you release.

Love,

Ron

Dear Friend,

It's important that you find a positive way to have memories of the source of your grief. You may be grieving a person or a pet. Love is the reason we grieve. It's not unusual for some people to be angry at the person or pet for leaving them through death. A "normal" person (whatever that means), may not understand you being angry at the source of your grief. Abandonment is how this feeling is described. The false premise is that the source of your grief chose to leave you. Children suffer from this most often but it's not unusual for adults to suffer from it also.

Not many people choose to die unless the pain from suffering is just so great that death is a welcomed escape. I don't know how much pain my wife was in before she died but I know she lived as long as she could for me and my daughter. Her doctor told me after my wife died that my wife told her that she was living for us. She lived two years beyond what the doctor expected. I never questioned why she died because I saw every day that she had a strong will to live.

I allow myself to remember our good times together. The good memories sustain me. I focus on the good times and I'm grateful that I could help her during the not so good times. Love is the source of grief and the more love you had the more grief you're going to have. I embrace the memories. I resented people telling me, "she'll always be with you." The fact was that she isn't her physically and I didn't want to hear that. As time passed I learned to embrace that statement and know that when I still myself she is with me through my memories.

Good memories can help us get through the grieving process.

Love,

Ron

Dear Friend,

One of the things I have begun to realize is that my wife wouldn't want me to be immobilized by grief. She willed herself to live beyond what the doctors said she would live. She did that to keep me and my daughter from grieving her. If I allow myself to be immobilized by her loss I'm disrespecting her. In my early days of loss I would wake up in the morning missing her. I wanted everything to return to the way it was. That was me being selfish. I didn't consider her journey through pain and discomfort. I didn't consider the losses she was enduring. I wanted her to protect me from losing her despite the fact that she was not well.

Once I embraced the idea that she was in a better place without pain and discomfort I could begin to heal. The "why me" attitude was replaced by a peace that came from knowing that she didn't have to wake up every day suffering in ways I never knew. Your journey through grief may not be specifically like mine but loss is loss. The specifics don't matter, the fact is you have suffered a loss. Your loss may have come suddenly and unexpectedly. You may have watched your loved one suffer over a period of time. The circumstances of the loss don't matter. What matters is that we suffered loss and we're trying to navigate through the grief process.

I read once that some people can't move from grief to the acceptance of loss because they feel like they had unfinished business with the source of their loss. You can never make up for loss moments and the only way you can move forward is to let go. Being angry with yourself is natural. The "what if's" come into our minds. In most cases there is nothing you can do. You can't go back in time. You can reflect on positive time spent with the source of your grief. The most common problem is not feeling like you had a chance to say goodbye or show the person what they meant to you. It's very likely the person knew how you felt but even if you could've said or done more it's in the past now. You have to pull yourself up and move forward. It's not easy but the first step is learning to forgive yourself.

Love,

Ron

Dear Friend,

One of the things you don't want to allow yourself to do is fall into denial. As painful as it is you must face the fact that you have lost a loved one. There are days I expect my wife to come into a room or say something to me and then I quickly realize that she's not ever coming back. These are healthy moments of grief. It becomes unhealthy for you when you don't acknowledge that the source of your grief is gone. Talking to your source of grief can be comforting. It can be a way of invoking their spirit into your life. Expecting them to answer you or physically be with you is not healthy and if you continue down that path you will find yourself in poor physical or mental health. There is no shame in seeking out counseling from someone who can guide you through the acceptance process. Seeking counseling is an act of strength not weakness. It takes a strong person to admit they need help. Sometimes we need to just say things openly and hear ourselves say them to confront the problem. A counselor can help you navigate through the difficult waters of depression which is the most difficult problem you'll face.

Depression early in the grieving process is normal. How long you stay in that stage of grief is what takes it from healthful to unhealthy. A lot of men find it difficult to get out of denial because little boys are discouraged from facing grief or hurt. The learned behavior is to ignore it and eventually it will go away. We're taught to "play through the pain" or "walk it off." That's denial disguised as strength. The longer you deny you're in pain the longer your recovery will be. You must breathe and grieve.

Love,

Ron

Dear Friend,

Sometimes grief hits us unexpectedly. A song, a picture, a movie or several other triggers may cause us to break down. Once again, this is nothing to be ashamed of. I have been going about my daily routine when I'm suddenly overcome with grief. I have no warning, no idea it's coming but wham—there it is. What I try to do is focus on the good memory behind the trigger. The trigger is based on a happy time usually so I force myself to focus on the positive and not allow the negative to overtake my emotions.

If you live in the same place you and your loved one lived in or go to restaurants you went to, or patronize businesses that you use to, there will be triggers. A familiar fragrance, a familiar song, a favorite movie, a favorite TV show and a myriad of other things will serve as triggers. You'll never be prepared for triggers, how could you be? After forty-nine years together my wife and I had so many things we shared that it's impossible for me not to have several triggers any given day. My way of surviving these triggers is to dwell on the good times we had rather than think about the fact we won't be able to experience those things together again.

Don't get the feeling that this process is easy. Triggers can be overwhelming each time you experience the same one so you should expect similar reactions to each trigger. I have to will myself to make it through every emotional challenge. I have learned to take on each challenge one day at a time. I get stronger with each day and refuse to allow myself to go backwards with my progress.

So, just know that each time you face a trigger you can focus on seeing the good things related to the trigger. Don't see the glass half empty when it's actually half full.

Love,

Ron

Dear Friend,

Loneliness is a natural by-product of grief. As I said in a previous letter, you may be fine when family and loved ones are around but suddenly be thrown into loneliness and despair once everyone leaves. You may be sitting in a room where you and your loved one sat or you may suddenly be sleeping alone in the bed the two of you shared, Whatever the case may be, loneliness comes in the quiet moments. If you live alone waking up to start your day may be your loneliest time.

Loneliness is normal and is to be expected. You may discover yourself talking to your loved one about something you know that they would be interested in and then discover they're not there. This happens to everyone at some point. The first thing people think to themselves is that they are "crazy." I'm not talking about being insane,

I'm talking about the description people use for an unexplainable reaction. Don't beat yourself up, move on. If you have family reach out to them at those times you and your loved one interacted. Call a friend, use social media, take on a new activity, interact with church or community members. Find something to do to keep yourself busy. You're not trying to forget or replace your loved one, you're simply trying to combat loneliness in a positive way.

A busy mind can combat loneliness. This book is a result of me writing letters to my wife. Writing is an activity that you do alone but being alone doesn't mean that you're lonely. Being lonely is in some cases a choice. You may have decided to cut yourself off from others. That is self imposed destructive loneliness. You're choosing loneliness over interacting with people. Sometimes it may be because you still have crying spells or times of sadness. Get over yourself, everyone who knows about your loss knows you're going to have periods of sadness. Men especially have difficulty with this because "real men don't cry." Real men who don't cry can have strokes or heart attacks because they refuse to release. Choosing loneliness over allowing people to see your pain is unhealthy physically and mentally.

Loneliness does not have to be your new normal. There are many groups that are designed to give people who have suffered loss an opportunity to get out and mingle with others. If you belong to a religious community, reach out. If you have a YMCA, gym or community center explore their offerings. Swim, play ping pong, work in a food pantry, answer phones or do clerical work. Bottom line, do something that will keep your mind busy and loneliness will be forced to fight for a spot in your life.

Love,

Ron

Dear Friend,

In a previous letter I mentioned that anger and resentment may creep in. This happens when you allow "why me" to fill your thoughts and go unchecked. Things happen in life that we can never understand. A line I remember from a movie is "why me?" The answer the person received was "why not you?" My take on that is good things and bad things happen to everybody. Do you ask why me when you receive the good? Probably not, you receive your good fortune and move on. So, if you move on in acceptance of the good, conversely, you must move on in acceptance of the bad.

It's natural to feel anger and resentment over a loss at first while in the shock stage but as time goes on we must learn to release the anger and resentment. There are people who have lost their religion because they were angry with God.

They resent that God allowed their loved one to die and they become overcome with anger. For a fleeting moment this is normal, we have to blame someone for the loss. Some people actually get angry with their loved one for leaving them. Some people aren't even aware that they are harboring that kind of anger.

It's difficult to confront the source of your anger. It means facing your loss and the changes in your life head on. In order to get beyond this point in your grief you must confront the anger and resentment. Identify the source and then work on ways to get beyond it. There's no time line for this process. Since no two people grieve the same way no two people are going to recover from grief in the same length of time. Some people who seemingly recover from grief quickly may not have really recovered from grief. They may have pushed it away in their mind in a way that may manifest itself some day in a negative way mentally and/or physically.

Don't put yourself on a recovery schedule, there is no schedule. You must confront your anger and resentment head on if you want to return to a functional life. Yes, this may have been totally unexpected, you may feel robbed of a life you thought you would have, you may resent the fact that you're left alone to find your way through this but you can come out of it with work. The first step of fighting a problem is to accurately identify the problem. Identify the cause of your anger and resentment and address it.

Love,

Ron

Dear Friend,

Because of finances, you may be forced to move or give up some of your possessions. This can be a blessing in disguise. It may free you of difficult memories and give you a chance to forge ahead. Some things aren't good or bad, they're just different. Don't assign labels of good or bad on events. Sometimes things just happen. That may sound simplified and maybe it is but the fact is, life goes on.

Finances may suddenly be cut in half because of the loss of a spouse but so are expenses. You have to come to grips with the "new normal." Your lifestyle is going to change with a loss. All of your expenses with the exception of your housing costs or car note will be cut in half. When formulating your new life plan, finances will play a significant part. Working on your budget can be helpful for you. Your mind will have something to keep it busy and not allow you to be overcome by your sense of loss. Should you be forced to move into more affordable housing you will be leaving a place wrapped up in memories. Emotionally you will be on a roller coaster. There will be sadness leaving memories behind and excitement and new energy as you move into a new life. How you allow yourself to view the new challenge will shape your recovery. The bottom line is that you can't stay in that emotional space, you must move forward.

Love,

Ron

Dear Friend,

When we are faced with death our bodies can go through physical distress. Stress and grief can take a severe physical strain on the human body. Using the teapot metaphor again, if you allow the pressure to build and go unchecked stress will attack your most vulnerable parts. You may have back pain, stomach distress, high blood pressure or heart problems. You may consult a physician to describe your physical problems but if they don't know the source of your problem they will only be acting on the symptoms and not the source.

If you have physical distress and contact a doctor it's important that you share with the doctor what you have gone through emotionally. That way the doctor can treat the physical manifestation of the stress and the underlying issues. It's important that you're open and honest with the doctor. The only way for you to get help is to seek help.

As soon as you address your physical distress your mental and emotional issues can be taken care of. You most likely won't be aware of what's going on with your body and your symptoms won't necessarily match a particular problem. Stress illnesses imitate real problems and disguise the source problem. Once again, this is why you must be open and frank with the doctor. Some people are afraid to talk to the doctor openly because they think the doctor may feel as though they are losing their mind. It's important to know that doctors don't make judgements like that and you're not the first or only person to go through stress related illnesses. The first step to fixing a problem is to admit that there is a problem.

Love,

Ron

Dear Friend,

Memories can be a double-edged sword. Most memories bring back thoughts of happy times that evoke sadness because we suddenly experience a sense of loss. It's important at these times to focus on the good parts of the memories. What makes this memory so special? Allow yourself to submerge in the beauty of the time of the memory and will yourself to let go of any sense of loss. Two opposing things can't occupy your thoughts at the same time. Don't allow yourself to go down the path to sadness. Remember a shared smile or laugh. Think about the sounds, the smells and the beauty of things around the memory.

When dealing with memories you have to consciously work at finding the good. Your subconscious will take over if you don't actively work to think about the good and close out the bad. Like everything else about grief, this isn't easy. When grieving it is much easier to succumb to sadness than it is to find happiness. Happiness exists in memories even if the memory is about the funeral or death. Memories are rooted in love and love is rooted in good. If you didn't care so much about the source of your grief you wouldn't feel such a sense of loss. This is the other side of the sword. This side cuts through the grief and allows the joy to come out. In Psalms 30:5 from the Bible it says, "Weeping may endure the night but JOY cometh in the morning!"

Free your mind and allow yourself to feel joy! Sometimes we feel guilty if we experience joy and happiness while in the middle of grief—don't! Being joyful of the memories for time shared is a good thing and is a way for you to climb out of the pit of grief and start to live again.

Love,

Ron

Dear Friend,

Once again I want to remind you that expressing emotion is a good thing. Tears cleanse the soul. Going back to the teapot analogy, emotions allow the mind and body to release. Tears are a major part of the release but crying has a stigma that won't allow you to use tears as a way to release. Think about this, by suppressing your tears you're suppressing your release. That's like closing a dam when the river is swollen. The water needs to go somewhere and if you don't release it the water is going to back up and do great damage. If you have ever seen a flood caused by water not being able to find a release you have a visual of how the suppression of your emotions affects your body. You may not see it or recognize it early on but the toll that suppressing emotions takes on the body is great. You may not be able to focus. You may slip into a depressed state. You may develop headaches or stomach problems. These symptoms are the body crying out to you to release. I have no problem crying. If men don't cry I lost my man card a long time ago. This is not to suggest that women don't have difficulty crying, some do. If crying is linked to strength then crying is a display of weakness. As this letter explains, crying actually helps the body regain or maintain its strength.

We are emotional beings. We feel joy and sadness; pain and pleasure; distress and relief. For every emotion there is an equal and opposite emotion. Free will gives us the opportunity to choose which end of the emotional pendulum we will swing on.

Choosing wisely prevents us from slipping into dark places from which it is difficult to escape.

Love,

Ron

Dear Friend,

Nothing prepares you for the first time you have to refer to yourself as a widow or widower. Filling out forms becomes a source of grief each time you fill one out. I was married for 44 years so two thirds of my life I filled out "married." I defined myself as a married man and then suddenly I wasn't.

Calling myself a widower still shocks my system. For a lot of people this seemingly benign answer is a real source of grief. Like everything else in order to overcome this you have to identify the problem and work your way through it. I had to figure out why I was so affected by this simple exercise of filling out a form. What I discovered was I had for so many years defined myself as a married man and now suddenly I had a title I didn't want thrust upon me.

As I worked through it I discovered that I was the same person and this wasn't better or worse, it was just different. That was my breakthrough. I found my "new" title and it was okay because it reminded me that I was lucky to have had someone in my life for so long we had defined ourselves as a married couple. I had no choice in selecting my new title but I did have a choice of accepting it. Accepting it helps me move beyond that stage of my grief.

Hello, I'm Ron and I'm a widower.

Love,

Ron

Dear Friend,

Sometimes grief causes us to want to withdraw from being around people. It's easier to withdraw than to let others see our pain. This may work in the short term but what you're actually doing is hiding from your problem. Telling yourself that you're grieving alone because you don't want to bring loved ones and friends down is the lie you tell yourself to justify your actions.

It may seemingly be affective for a while but eventually you'll find yourself alone and possibly more depressed. Interacting with people is a way of keeping yourself from falling deeper into depression. You may find yourself overeating, drinking or doing drugs to "take off the edge." In the end, grief may be the least of your problems. There's something about having to put on a happy face to greet the day that actually causes you to have a happy face. Knowing that you actually have to face people makes you have to confront your underlying problems.

Depression causes you to want to withdraw. Once again, this is normal for the early stages of the grieving process but as time goes on it's not good for your mental health. We are not meant to be alone. Watch babies and toddlers. They gravitate towards others when they here sounds from other children or adults. One of the ways psychologists test children is to observe how they react during social interactions. It's literally in the human DNA to join their tribe. That doesn't change as we get older so isolating yourself is not normal behavior.

The expression "it takes a village " encompasses natural human instincts and behavior. Your "village" will reach out to you if they know you're in pain. It's your responsibility to respond to them. You may not want to reach out to others but you shouldn't reject their overtures to you.

Love,

Ron

Dear Friend,

Panic is another part of grieving. We panic about finances, we panic about being alone, we panic about household management, we panic about having to face the world alone and we panic about what the future holds for us moving alone. Each of these things can be overwhelming when faced alone but combined can be the cause of deep anxiety. Anxiety is a form of panic and is also an indication of depression.

Most people think depression is sadness but depression is multifaceted. Depression and anxiety usually manifest at the same time during the grieving process. There are people who are depressed who don't cry or exhibit any signs of what most of us perceive as sadness. Some people can't cry which is a healthy part of releasing so they become anxious, confused and panicky. As I've said before, this is normal. Panic is the mind's way of telling you that you have a problem that needs to be addressed. If you don't stop and listen a panic attack demands that you stop and take note that there's something wrong.

I have a friend who ignored all of the signs that something was wrong until a panic attack caused her to go to the floor and curl up into the fetal position. Her father couldn't pull her out of her anxiety attack for hours until he brought in professional help. Fortunately, after weeks of therapy she faced the pain of grief and change that caused her problem. Now she is able to socialize and help others face their grief before it causes them to experience what she experienced. It wasn't easy for her but she was able to face the root of the problem.

Love,

Ron

Dear Friend,

Sometimes people worry about being happy while grieving. It's okay to be happy during the time you're grieving. There's no reason to feel guilty should you have feelings of joy and happiness while grieving. You can have mood swings between joy and sadness while grieving and it's a normal part of the grieving process. You can go between laughing at a good memory to crying about the same.

The key is that life for you must go on. Your loved one wouldn't want you to waste away into I'll health grieving them. Your "new normal" may mean that you have to adjust to going between joy and happiness combined with grief and sorrow. The important thing for you is to not get bogged down in grief or depression. Accept the joy that comes in the morning.

Love,

Ron

Dear Friend,

There may be some days that you have to force yourself out of bed. In the early days of your loss this can be expected. Trying to find balance and a way to face the day without the one you loss can be very difficult. The more you force yourself to move on the more natural it will become. Conversely, the more you withdraw and stay in bed the more natural that will become. You must allow yourself to return to "normal" carrying out daily routines and interacting with others. At first, family, friends and associates will be guarded interacting with you for fear they may say of do something that triggers you into sorrow or a crying spell.

This is all normal as you start to adjust yourself emotionally. Others will follow your lead. Accept shoulders to cry on, ears to listen and arms to steady you.

Eventually you'll once again be able to stand alone but for now, accept help. Get up each day ready to face the challenges even though you're going through difficult times. It won't necessarily be better or worse but it will be different.

Being different is okay. In my case, after so many years of facing challenges with my partner beside me I suddenly had to start each day alone.

The first thing I had to do was adjust myself to the point that I would be facing life without my wife but I had it within me to carry on. That first step meant getting out of bed.

Love,

Ron

Dear Friend,

Sometimes grief disguises itself as an illness. This usually happens when you don't want to acknowledge your grief so your body has to find an excuse to shut you down. Stress illnesses are common for grieving people. You try to trudge on but your body suddenly shuts down.

This is a lot more normal than you might expect. The conscious mind refuses to grieve so the subconscious mind takes over. This is a psychosomatic episode. That doesn't mean you have a mental problem, it means that the mind has taken over to protect itself and your body. You consciously won't acknowledge the need to stop and openly grieve but your brain shifts into survival mode. No medicine can help the physical manifestation no matter how strong the medicine is, your mind controls when the physical problem clears up. Usually, once your body shuts down your mind begins to go through the grieving process. This may be a crying spell or just a sluggish feeling. Whatever it is you must let it run its course. Some people try to self medicate with alcohol or drugs but self medication doesn't help. The mind just needs to heal itself and that healing means facing the problem. Once again, the hardest thing for most people to do is to be patient and allow the process to play out.

Love,

Ron

Dear Friend,

While you're grieving life and death go on. One of the most difficult things you will experience is losing someone close while you're grieving. There's never a good time to lose someone but if it happens while you're grieving all of your feelings of loss come back. The idea of attending a funeral is challenging. Some people can't go to funerals and others can. There's no right or wrong, you have to listen to your emotions and decide if attending a funeral is going to be a problem for your emotional or mental health. There will be people who will try to "guilt you" into attending a funeral but calling the people who lost someone or visiting them before the funeral may be best for you. If you feel overwhelmed during a visit you can leave but if you become overwhelmed at the funeral you may feel required to stay.

There will be some who have never experienced grief who won't understand what you're going through. You can't allow them to force you into a situation that you know won't be good for you. Being open and honest with them will help you and possibly help them understand. Be prepared for them not to understand and make your decision based on what you feel is best for you.

Love,

Ron

Dear Friend,

As I'm writing this book the Coronavirus (Covid-19) is taking a lot of lives. Some families are losing multiple members in a short period of time. One of the big problems with losing people during a pandemic is that families aren't allowed to visit or spend time with their loved ones. This makes the loss even more difficult. Not being able to see your loved one during their final days means you don't get to say goodbye. You don't get closure because of the unspoken things you wanted to say. Just because you didn't get to say them to the person while they were alive doesn't mean you can't say them. Saying those things to your loved one is a way for you to release. Write them down and read them at the grave, speak it in your house, talk to them while driving, express your feelings as a release and internal cleansing. Let it out, don't suppress your feelings.

As I've said in previous letters, don't let this fester inside you. Grief can literally eat at you from the inside physically and mentally. There are so many illnesses that are caused by grieving. Ulcers, high blood pressure, heart trouble, depression and anxiety among other things can develop as a direct result of grief.

Love,

Ron

Dear Friend,

Holidays are some of the most difficult times for those of us who are grieving. Holidays are filled with good memories and bring back good times together. It's easy to give in to sorrow but if you allow yourself to relive your memories you'll discover that the holidays are actually filled with great memories. If you get past the initial pain from the memories, memories of the good times will bring you through the sorrow.

Don't allow yourself to withdraw into sadness and dread holidays, let yourself remember the beautiful times spent together. Rather than weeping during the holidays try hard to allow yourself to be filled with joy.

Love,

Ron

Dear Friend,

When you're grieving all of your senses can become triggers for sadness. A familiar smell or fragrance, a sound, music, pictures or visuals, a familiar food or drink. Some of these triggers may surprise you and wash over your body. These are sometimes the things that lead to unexpected crying spells. This is normal when grieving. As I've said before, in some cases everything that made you happy as a couple, a close relative or a friend don't disappear or stop when the person dies. You will continue to experience these things, you just won't be able to share them with your loved one. You may even catch yourself talking to your loved one about something you've experienced until you suddenly remember that they are not there. The most difficult thing that hits you is the realization that you'll never experience these things with your loved one again. It's important that when this happens you focus your attention on why these triggers affect you. The reason they affect you is that they are wrapped up in good memories. Don't allow yourself to be so affected by your loss that you forget the good times. Each trigger that affects you negatively can be turned around as a positive trigger. Allow yourself to smile through the good and not be negatively affected by the bad. The reason you hurt so much from the triggers is because they represent good or happy times.

Love,

Ron

Dear Friend,

It's a natural part of grieving in the early stages to want to avoid social gatherings or family gatherings without your loved one. If you have good friends, family members or church members, they will try to pull you back into their circle. A month after my wife died, my brother and his wife were celebrating their 50th wedding anniversary. I didn't know if I would be able to attend. My daughter and I decided that we would go.

When I got to the celebration most of the people who were in attendance had attended my wife's funeral a month before. To my pleasant surprise I was able to attend and not be overcome by sorrow. In fact, I was able to speak on the program and share good memories.

When I woke up the next morning I felt a lightness I hadn't felt since my wife passed. I experienced my favorite scripture come to life. I felt Joy! Had I not gone I don't think I would've felt the release I felt.

Love,

Ron

Dear Friend,

"Do not grieve, for the joy of the Lord is your strength." This is from Nehemiah 8:10. This passage speaks to you even if you're not religious. The emotions that fuel grief are the same emotions that once fueled joy. You will need to find your way back to joy if you want to recover from grief. That may sound difficult but when a memory comes to mind and you feel a pang of grief let the memory play itself out. Initially you will feel the pain of grief. If you let the memory continue you will find yourself begin to experience the joy that caused the memory to come to mind. Even if it's a memory from a dark experience love can be found at its center.

Because you loved the one you lost you cared about their pain or misfortune. You may feel bad because you couldn't save them from pain and suffering. If you allow the

memory to play out you may discover that just being with them you may have helped them more than you initially thought. There may be a look they gave you or something they said that you overlooked in the moment that you recognize as you reflect that will help you recover. If you don't allow yourself to get to the conclusion of the memory you may not have closure. One of the worst parts of grieving is the feeling that you didn't do enough. If you replay the experience you will probably discover that you did everything humanly possible.
Love,

Ron

Dear Friend,

By now you should be experiencing a degree of acceptance. This is not acceptance of the loss, it's the acceptance of the fact that life must go on. Take a moment to assess where you are and how far you've come. If you have meditated on the things you have gotten from these letters, you should've discovered an inner strength you weren't aware that you possessed at the beginning of the book. You should be beyond the many stages of grief and be ready to start living again.

This does not mean that you won't still feel the loss, it simply means that you should've discovered coping mechanisms. This journey has been difficult but hopefully you have found your balance as you've faced your loss.

Love,

Ron

Dear Friend,

As we near the conclusion of our 30 day journey, it's time for some affirmations.

1) I am stronger than I thought I was at the beginning of this journey.
2) I don't have to fear tomorrow.
3) If I allow myself to feel joy, I can heal from within.
4) Living my life does not mean I have forgotten my loved one.
5) I will always feel the love I have for my loved, that will never end.
6) My life is different, not necessarily better or worse but it is different.

As you affirm these things allow yourself to release them.

Love,

Ron

Dear Friend,

Releasing the grief does not mean that you are "abandoning" your loved one. It means that your love for them has grown into another way. Physical contact may no longer be possible but that doesn't mean that they are no longer in your heart or with you in your memories. Should you enjoy the company of others it's not a betrayal of them.

Moving on with your life is fulfilling your purpose in life. Your loved one would want you to find joy. Allowing yourself to open up to others is part of that. Once you can laugh and smile with others without feeling guilt, you are finding your way back. Does this mean that you won't feel sorrow, no. It means that you've found balance.

Love,

Ron

Dear Friend,

You've seen me write about balance and joy throughout this book. Balance means being able to go about your daily activities without being depressed or anxious. If by this point after reflecting on what you've read you still feel depressed or anxious, please reach out to a professional counselor and let them guide you through the healing process.

What it probably means is that you're dealing with problems or issues that weren't covered in these letters. This book is not intended to be an end of grieving for everyone, it's intended to help you recognize and address the grieving process. Your next step may be to reach out for one on one help. Hopefully, these letters have helped you realize what needs to be addressed.

Love,

Ron

Dear Friend,

Grief is an ongoing problem. It just becomes less difficult to understand and address over time. You shouldn't feel at the end of this book that you've been "cured" of grieving. Even after going through counseling you may need to follow up with your counselor to "fine tune" some of your coping mechanisms. Once again, you're not alone having to do this, there's nothing wrong with you should you need to reach out until you feel balanced. Life without your loved one will never be the same but that doesn't mean you can't go on living.

Love,

Ron

Made in the USA
Columbia, SC
14 February 2024